Living Well With Hemochromatosis

A Handbook on Diet, Iron Overload Treatments and Protective Supplements

Ralph Catalase, M.S. Nutrition

ISBN-13: 978-1482741537
ISBN-10: 1482741539

DISCLAIMER

This information within this book contains information on supplements, studies and treatment protocols. Do NOT construe this as medical advice. Medical advice can only be given by a licensed professional who has had a chance to personally observe you and who understands your condition, position and objectives. The information presented here is not intended to replace the attention or advice of a physician or other health care professional. It talks about health issues in general for a 'statistical' user, not you as a specific user, and is not referring to your specific healthcare issues. Anyone who wishes to embark on any dietary, drug, exercise, supplement or other lifestyle change intended to prevent or treat a specific disease or condition should first consult with and seek clearance from a qualified healthcare practitioner. Please call a health professional immediately if you think you may be ill.

This information has not been reviewed or approved by the FDA. It is provided under First Amendment rights for educational and communication purposes only, and should not be construed as personal medical advice. Therefore, this information and any products presented along with it should be used only to inform yourself about available choices in conjunction with consultation of a healthcare professional. No actions should be taken based solely on the contents of this book alone. Its information should NOT be interpreted as a recommendation for a specific treatment plan, nor should this information be used in place of the medical opinion of a qualified health care professional. It is NOT intended to replace, supplant, or augment a consultation with a doctor or health professional regarding the reader's/user's own medical care. In the event you choose not to consult with a healthcare professional and self-diagnose and/or self-treat yourself, using this information or products, neither this author or publisher can, nor will, assume any responsibilities for the results.

Anyone who wishes to embark on any dietary, drug, exercise, or other lifestyle change intended to treat or prevent a specific condition should first consult with their doctor; readers who fail to consult appropriate health authorities assume the full risk of any injuries. The author and publisher disclaim and all liability for injury or damages that could result from the use of information obtained from this book. No matter what testimonials say, no matter what studies say, no matter what opinion says, even the most benign product and/or protocol may have rare negative consequences for you personally. The authors and publisher are not responsible for any errors or omissions in this book, or the use of the information within. The information published within is only as current as the day the book was produced. The protocols raise many issues that are subject to change as new data emerge. None of the treatment protocols featured within guarantee or promise a cure for Hemochromatosis.

CONTENTS

TO YOUR HEALTH

For all individuals suffering from hemochromatosis and iron overload illnesses, I hope this small book sufficiently educates you about the characteristics of your condition. It provides enough dietary guidelines so that you can reduce your tendency to absorb iron through natural means, teaches you how to protect your liver and other internal organs through the use of nutritional supplements, and might even help you cut down on the number of necessary phlebotomies or chelations you must undergo each year.

Please remember that hemochromatosis is a lifelong condition. You can reduce your iron overload by eating low iron foods, by refraining from eating foods that increase your iron uptake, and by eating foods with meals that bind iron or which naturally chelate it out of the body. If you remember these basic strategies, and take the relevant nutritional supplements to help protect and strengthen your internal organs, you can and will live very well with hemochromatosis and hardly notice any lifestyle changes at all.

1
WHAT IS HEMOCHROMATOSIS?

Hemochromatosis is an inherited genetic condition that causes the body to absorb and store too much iron in the tissues. The condition is also called "iron overload" or "iron storage overload" disease. It is dangerous because while iron is an essential component of the hemoglobin in our red blood cells that enables these cells to transport oxygen, in its unbound form it also has a destructive nature that accelerates the oxidation or "rusting" of body tissues. This is particularly harmful to internal organs, such as the liver.

Of all the genetic disorders, hemochromatosis is the most common, and routinely affects over one million people in just the United States alone. This means that approximately one million Americans per year are overloading with excess iron – twice as many as those who suffer from the problem of iron deficiency anemia. Additionally, hereditary hemochromatosis is also the most commonly inherited liver disease in Europe.

Hereditary hemochromatosis (HH), also known as genetic hemochromatosis (GH), is triggered by a defective gene that causes one amino acid to be substituted for another in a protein. About 1 in 127 to 1 in 270 patients inherit the gene from both parents to get the disease; the gene is prevalent in Hispanics and in about 20% of people of northern European stock.

In terms of total figures, approximately 33 million Americans (10% of the population) are carriers for hemochromatosis but don't know it, and only a minority of these carriers actually manifests the disease.

Usually, most people have inherited the gene from an ancient ancestor living centuries ago … in particular, ancestors of Irish, German, English, Scottish, Welsh origin. A person who inherits two identical genes ("homozygous") will always pass on the disease to their offspring.

The physical basis of hemochromatosis is simple: the intestines absorb twice as much iron from food as normal, and thus excess iron slowly builds up in the body tissues. Many cases of hemochromatosis go undiagnosed because doctors and patients are unaware of the condition and don't know what to look for. The early symptoms include fatigue, sore joints and frequent infections, so they are easy to mistake for other conditions.

Nevertheless, as the excess iron builds up in the organs – especially in the liver, heart, spleen, and pancreas – it tends to destroy cells. Some people have no outward symptoms whatsoever until the condition matures in mid-age, at which time they may have 200 times the normal levels of iron!

That is when it can really cause problems.

Joint pain and sore joints are the most common early complaints of people who have hemochromatosis. Other common symptoms include fatigue, weakness and lack of energy. There can also be a loss of libido/sex drive, abdominal pains and swelling, and various heart problems, such as heart flutters. There can also be a history of frequent infections, skin bronzing or hair loss.

The symptoms tend to occur in men between the ages of 30 and 50 and in women over age 50 after they stop menstruating. Women are less at risk than men for iron buildup because of the fact that they lose iron during their monthly menstruation. However, many people have no symptoms at all when they are first diagnosed.

If the condition persists without being diagnosed, by the time someone is fifty or sixty with iron build-up, the organs may have literally "rusted inside" and will definitely show damage of some sort. Iron is nature's rusting ("oxidation") agent, even inside our body, and the buildup of excess iron levels within is one of the ways by which our body becomes oxidized, and therefore subject to premature aging.

The excess iron inside our bodies is harmful because it is a catalyst for the generation of free radical activity, and free radicals have been identified as an underlying cause of cancer, atherosclerosis, liver cirrhosis, neurological disease, and other aging-related disorders.

Liver cirrhosis, liver cancer, heart failure, diabetes, arthritis are all possibilities for hemochromatosis sufferers if the excess iron builds up to cause tissue damage. The damage to one's liver and pancreas is especially dangerous because the harmful results can be permanent. One of the side effects of hemochromatosis is a yellowish skin complexion and diabetes like symptoms that give HH the name "bronze diabetes." Other possibilities from hemochromatosis include an enlarged liver (hepatomegaly), cirrhosis (liver scarring), and spleen enlargement (splenomegaly).

The following are some of the common symptoms of hereditary hemochromatosis (HH):

- Chronic fatigue and weakness
- Sore or aching joints, especially in the knuckle and first joint of the first and second fingers
- Frequent infections (colds, flu and other signs of weakened immune system)

- Abdominal pain/swelling
- Red palms
- Impotence – low libido (males) – sterility - infertility
- Cirrhosis of the liver (with or without history of alcohol use)
- Liver cancer (with or without history of alcohol use)
- An enlarged liver or other liver disease
- Arthritis or joint pain (or joint replacement)
- Slightly elevated liver enzymes
- "Bronze diabetes" – abnormal gray or bronze discoloration of the skin
- Early menopause/irregular menses
- Darkening of the skin without exposure to the sun
- Always feeling "cold"
- Hair loss, loss of body hair
- Weight loss
- Cancer
- Headaches
- Hypothyroidism (thyroid deficiency)
- Adrenal gland damage
- Heart irregularities/heart failure/heart attack (particularly in younger men)

The screening to check for hemochromatosis involves multiple tests rather than just one blood test. Doctors need to measure a number of different factors to determine if you suffer from hemochromatosis. A skilled hematologist, who is an expert at blood conditions, is often the best professional to consult concerning your blood iron levels.

For instance, "low iron" on one blood test does NOT rule out hemochromatosis. Hemochromatosis often goes undiagnosed because it can show up on a blood test through a low hemoglobin level, just as does iron depletion. A person can also actually be anemic and still be suffering from iron overload hemochromatosis!

Therefore, because the symptoms can be diverse and vague and can mimic the symptoms of many other conditions, and because blood tests can be misinterpreted, hemochromatosis often goes undiagnosed and untreated.

Frankly, many doctors just don't think to test for it. Instead, doctors most often focus on the conditions caused by hemochromatosis— arthritis, liver disease, fibromyalgia, chronic fatigue syndrome, irritable bowel syndrome, heart disease, or diabetes—rather than search for the underlying cause to find this condition.

Here's the good news. There are a number of solutions available for hemochromatosis when it's found. In addition, if the iron overload caused by hemochromatosis is diagnosed and treated before organ damage has occurred, a person can live a normal, healthy life.

In the next chapter, we'll talk about various screening tests available to confirm the condition.

2
MEDICAL SCREENING FOR HEMOCHROMATOSIS

Your physician (sometimes with the help of a hematologist) arrives at a definitive diagnosis of hereditary hemochromatosis (HH) based upon:

(1) Taking a thorough medical history (including questions about any family history of arthritis or unexplained liver disease and family heritage because of a possible genetic component).

(2) A physical examination.

(3) Various blood tests that measure the presence of iron overload.

(4) DNA genetic testing that searches for specific hemochromatosis mutations.

If your doctor suspects hereditary hemochromatosis, they will order a genetic blood test to look for the HFE mutation that is responsible for the disorder.

Let's talk about the standard blood tests first before we talk about the genetic testing...

Iron Blood Tests

As previously stated, hemochromatosis often goes undiagnosed because the condition – even though it is characterized by high iron levels in the body – sometimes shows up on a blood tests as low hemoglobin, which you also find in cases of iron depletion anemia. Hence a condition of too much iron may actually be hidden by blood work measurements that indicate deficient iron levels in the blood. Since doctors aren't trained to look for the condition but normally treat the symptoms of hemochromatosis as it affects various organs and body symptoms, it often escapes diagnosis.[1]

If you suspect hemochromatosis, blood tests for **serum iron, total iron binding capacity (TIBC)** and **serum transferrin** are good ways to begin the initial screening for hemochromatosis. Any blood testing lab can do these tests for you, and most doctors will order them for you without any problems.

Your doctor must specifically request an **iron series profile** on the lab requisition form otherwise all three of these specific tests might not be done. I cannot tell you the number of times I've advised people to get blood tests for specific markers only to find out later that only half of the requested measures were done.

You can also call Healthcheck USA (www.healthcheckusa.com) at 1-800-929-2044 to find a blood testing lab near you. Blood testing for a complete iron profile, which includes, serum iron, TIBC and serum ferritin and genetic test kits that you use at home are available from this company. Remember when asking your doctor for iron testing to mention all three tests by name, and also ask for copies of the reports. You should not have to do any testing on your own, but just ask your doctor to order all the relevant tests if you suspect the condition and he/she has not thought of it.

Also remember to take these blood tests in a fasting state, preferably in the morning, because that's when you will get the most accurate results. Over 50% of individuals have elevated serum iron levels after

---

[1] Acton RT, Barton JC, Casebeer L, et. al. "Survey of physician knowledge about hemochromatosis." *Genet Med.* 2002 May-Jun; 4(3):136-41.

eating, so if the tests are taken on a full stomach, the iron levels that are measured can be elevated even if there are no increased iron stores

Another good test is the **serum transferring receptor test,** but it is not yet available at most blood testing laboratories. If you suspect hemochromatosis, ask for these four tests which help screen for the condition:

- **Total Iron Binding Capacity** (TIBC) - measures how well your blood can transport iron
- **Serum Iron Test**
- **Serum Ferritin** - shows the level of iron in the liver
- **Serum transferring receptor** (not yet available at most laboratories)

Once your doctor has these tests he can start making some calculations, and then some preliminary conclusions.

The first calculation is to determine the "percent of saturation," also known as the "transferrin saturation" level. The transferrin saturation measure is calculated by dividing the serum iron results by the TIBC results and multiplying the fraction by 100 to arrive at a percentage.

$$\text{Transferrin Saturation} = 100 * \frac{\text{Serum Iron Concentration}}{\text{Total Iron Binding Capacity}}$$

There are various diagnostic cutoff levels for the levels of transferrin saturation and serum ferritin, which have varied across studies, that suggest hemochromatosis. In other words, doctors use different decision thresholds for transferrin saturation, serum ferritin level, and their combined results to diagnose hemochromatosis.

Here's how to interpret the figures.

A normal transferrin saturation measure is between 20% and 50%. Therefore, a transferrin saturation greater than 50% is a warning flag identifying people who may have excessive iron loading tendencies. That's a warning sign for hemochromatosis. Some doctors have proposed that the screening cutoff point should be 60% for males and 50% for women. Other doctors recommend a lower screening figure of 40%, too, which is a figure we'll focus on.

A percent of saturation figure greater than 40% and/or a serum ferritin greater than 150 ng/ml (>150 ng/mL) is a general set of looser measures that also suggest the condition, and we have to say "suggests" the condition because not all individuals having these measurements have hemochromatosis. That's why we still need to call this a "warning flag."

The initial screening levels for hemochromatosis, that suggest further investigation, are definitely still being argued about. I would rather err on the side of caution when various symptoms are present, and therefore would argue that the lower cutoff values seem more logical than the higher. The higher the levels, however, the higher the probability of true hemochromatosis and the lower the cutoff levels, the lower the probability of the condition.

In some medical studies, higher cutoff levels (transferrin saturation $\geq$ 62% and serum ferritin levels $\geq$ 500 µg/L) identified a subgroup of individuals in which *all of them* had hereditary hemochromatosis. A set of less stringent criteria (transferrin saturation $\geq$ 45% and serum ferritin levels > 200 µg/L) identified a group of individuals in which only 11.5% had hereditary hemochromatosis.[2,3,4]

---

[2] Baer DM, Simons JL, Staples RL, Rumore GJ, Morton CJ. "Hemochromatosis screening in asymptomatic ambulatory men 30 years of age and older." *Am J Med.* 1995; 98:464-8.

[3] Phatak PD, Sham RL, Raubertas RF, Dunnigan K, O'Leary MT, Braggins C, et al. "Prevalence of hereditary hemochromatosis in 16031 primary care patients." *Ann Intern Med.* 1998; 129:954-61.

[4] Niederau C, Niederau CM, Lange S, Littauer A, Abdel-Jalil N, Maurer M, et al. "Screening for hemochromatosis and iron deficiency in employees and

Basically, the **combination of an elevated transferrin saturation and an elevated serum ferritin level** are together extremely accurate for predicting hemochromatosis.[5]

Therefore, the screening criteria are not conclusive determinants of hemochromatosis, but only prompt one to next perform DNA tests that confirm the presence of the gene defects. After all, other factors can work to raise various blood iron figures, including the measurement of transferrin saturation.

The reason that transferrin saturation is preferred over serum ferritin when determining hemochromatosis is because it's a more sensitive and specific test than serum ferritin, which can become elevated for a large variety of reasons. Serum ferritin can also be normal in some cases of hemochromatosis, or greatly under report the amount of iron that has actually accumulated in the body.

Since we're looking for to help zero in on the easily missed condition of hemochromatosis, and since serum ferritin can be abnormally elevated in various conditions such as Gaucher's disease, congenital cataracts, rheumatoid arthritis, malignancies, hepatitis and liver injury or alcohol abuse, transferrin saturation is the best first measure to focus on when looking for hereditary hemochromatosis.

Individuals with a transferrin saturation level > 40% and serum ferritin > 150ng/mL are typically suffering from iron overload/excess iron storage in the body due to some reason, even if it is not due to hemochromatosis, and doctors will normally treat them with phlebotomies regardless of whether or not DNA test results confirm a hemochromatosis diagnosis.

Why?

---

primary care patients in Western Germany." *Ann Intern Med.* 1998; 128:337-45.
[5] Feldman: *Sleisenger & Fordtran's Gastrointestinal and Liver Disease, 6th ed.,* 1998, W. B. Saunders Company.

Because if someone is proven to have excess iron in their system then they are in danger of organ damage and premature death if the condition is left untreated. Therefore, they should undergo a series of phlebotomies in order to reduce the excessive iron levels in their body, and we'll discuss this and other options for reducing the body's iron stores in the next chapter.

What are the other iron measures that suggest hemochromatosis?

As seen in the chart below, the serum ferritin level will also usually be elevated in most patients with hemochromatosis.

SERUM	NORMAL	HEMOCHROMATOSIS
Transferrin Saturation (%)	20-50%	55-100%
Ferritin (ng/mL)		
* Males	20-200	300-3000
* Females	15-150	250-3000
Iron * mug/dL	60-180	180-300
* mumol/L	11-32	32-54

Genetic Tests

If these blood tests are abnormally high, then the next step to confirming a diagnosis is to perform a genetic test for the mutations in the HFE gene.[6] Typically, anywhere from 85-98% of patients with clinical iron overload will show the presence of the hemochromatosis mutations.

What is this expected mutation?

Hereditary (or genetic) hemochromatosis is mainly associated with a defect in a gene called *HFE* whose purpose is to help regulate the amount of iron we absorb from the foods we eat. There are two known important mutations in *HFE*, named Cys282Y and His63D, and DNA tests to confirm hemochromatosis look for these specific mutations.

The DNA gene testing that can confirm hemochromatosis must test for both HFE mutations (Cys282Y & His63D, also known as C282Y and H63D) and is called **HLA-H**, or more commonly the HFE or Hfe test. Remember that if you want these tests, you have to ask for these tests by name – the **Cys282Y and His63D mutation tests**.

Not all labs test for both hemochromatosis mutations so this should be the main question when considering lab tests. These genetic tests are commercially available and cost about $200.

Cys282Y is the most important defect to look for. When the Cys282Y abnormality is inherited from both parents, dietary iron is usually over-absorbed and hemochromatosis can result. His63D usually does cause a little increase in iron absorption, but a person with His63D from one parent and Cys282Y from the other will rarely develop hemochromatosis.

You must also understand that HLA-typing (the HFE test) is not the same as genetic DNA testing, so be sure not to get confused about some older forms of testing that many labs still offer. Rather, to confirm hemochromatosis you must be sure to ask for DNA testing by the specific name of the mutations: **cys282** (pronounced "siss two

---

[6] This gene is the result of a single base change in which tyrosine is substituted for cysteine at position 282 of the HFE protein (Cys282Y).

eighty two) and **his63** (pronounced "hiss sixty-three), and mention you're looking to confirm hemochromatosis to make sure you are getting the correct tests.

If the test results come back positive, then it's also important to test any of your children for the gene mutations so that you can assess their risks for hemochromatosis before any damage occurs. Early tests can help determine whether there is anyone else in the family who might be at risk for storing excessive iron in the future.

The solution?

Act now!

Liver Biopsy

A patient's physician may also want to test liver enzymes (usually they will be elevated due to some degree of liver dysfunction) and investigate the family history in order to confirm a diagnosis of the genetic disorder.

A liver biopsy can also show exactly how much excessive iron the liver is storing, and can reveal the extent of liver damage in advanced cases of hemochromatosis. Among other things, the liver biopsy is normally used to diagnose primary liver cancer, and liver cancer is a possible outcome of advanced hemochromatosis.

Depending on whether there is evidence of liver damage, your doctor may suggest a liver biopsy should be done to assess the damage to your liver. In a liver biopsy, a tiny piece of liver tissue is removed and examined under a microscope to reveal how much iron has accumulated in its cells. This determines whether the liver is damaged, and to what degree.

Liver biopsies are invasive procedures, and you can tell your doctor that a biopsy might not be necessary if you cite certain research.

You can point your doctor to a 1998 study in *Gastroenterology*[7] that examined 197 French hemochromatosis patients who had the Cys282Y homozygous gene. The purpose of the study was to determine if there were any noninvasive predictors of severe liver fibrosis, which is a complication usually involving cirrhosis.

The study found that simple biochemical and clinical blood variables -- **serum aspartate aminotransferase, serum ferritin**, and **hepatomegaly** -- were just as predictive as invasive liver biopsies except when making a diagnosis of severe fibrosis.

What were the results of this study, and others?

> It was derived in a French population and validated in a Canadian population. Only 1 of 105 patients (0.9%) with a ferritin level of 1000 µg/L or less had cirrhosis. In combination with a normal aspartate aminotransferase (AST) level and no hepatomegaly, 0 of 94 patients had cirrhosis. Findings in the validation population were similar. The more recent follow-up report[8] found that ferritin levels greater than 1000 µg/L, platelet counts less than 200 x 10^9 cells/L, and elevated AST levels led to a correct diagnosis of cirrhosis in 77% of the Canadian participants and in 90% of the French participants who were tested. Morrison and colleagues[9] found that patients with ferritin levels less than 1000 µg/L were unlikely to

---

[7] Guyader D, Jacquelinet C, Moirand R, Turlin B, Mendler MH, Chaperon J, et al. "Noninvasive prediction of fibrosis in C282Y homozygous hemochromatosis." *Gastroenterology.* 1998; 115:929-36.
[8] Beaton M, Guyader D, Deugnier Y, Moirand R, Chakrabarti S, Adams P. "Noninvasive prediction of cirrhosis in C282Y-linked hemochromatosis." *Hepatology.* 2002; 36:673-8.
[9] Morrison ED, Brandhagen DJ, Phatak PD, Barton JC, Krawitt EL, El-Serag HB, et al. "Serum ferritin level predicts advanced hepatic fibrosis among U.S. patients with phenotypic hemochromatosis." *Ann Intern Med.* 2003; 138:627-33. [PMID: 12693884].

have cirrhosis on liver biopsy (1 of 93 patients). These 3 studies strongly suggest that patients who are at high risk for hereditary hemochromatosis (homozygous C282Y mutation) with serum ferritin levels of 1000 μg/L or less are unlikely to have cirrhosis.[10]

Let's summarize this in English.

A rule to predict the presence of liver cirrhosis (liver damage sometimes caused by hemochromatosis) has already been developed and validated, and can help your doctor avoid the need for a biopsy. From this research, the following is the profile of an individual *unlikely* to have cirrhosis:

- Serum ferritin level < 1000 μg/L without hepatomegaly and
- Normal AST level

Individuals with a high probability of liver cirrhosis will typically show:

- Serum ferritin levels > 1000 μg/L
- Platelet counts < 200 x 10^9 cells/L, and
- Elevated AST levels

The earlier your diagnosis of hemochromatosis, the less your chances of ever needing a liver biopsy, which just serves to point out the importance of early screening for HH. If you must have a liver biopsy performed, ask your doctor to use ultrasound or CT to help guide the biopsy.

Patients at high risk for liver cancer because of hemochromatosis should be screened periodically with various blood tests[11] for the rest of their lives.

---

[10] http://www.annals.org/cgi/content/full/143/7/522?ck=nck
[11] Alpha fetoprotein and PIVKA-II.

The big take-away from all this is that hemochromatosis is not a diagnosis arrived at by just one test. First there are blood tests, and then genetic tests looking for the confirmation of gene mutations. Your physical condition is also taken into account.

If one is identified early enough, there are various treatments for hemochromatosis (phlebotomies) that do involve some mild discomfort and inconvenience, but an individual can live a long and normal life with these treatments.

Let's turn to the conventional treatments, and then the alternative treatments that can help with this condition.

3
TRADITIONAL HEMOCHROMATOSIS IRON OVERLOAD TREATMENTS

Because hemochromatosis can adversely affect a number of organs in the body, treatment is usually handled by any number of professionals including a hepatologist (liver disorder specialist), gastroenterologist (specialist in digestive disorders), and hematologist (specialist in blood disorders).

Several other medical specialists may also help in treating the condition including a cardiologist (because of the heart problems), endocrinologist, or rheumatologist (because of joint problems). Internists and family practitioners can also treat the disease.

What is the main treatment for hemochromatosis?

Hemochromatosis is conventionally treated through **phlebotomy treatments**, also known as blood letting or donating blood.

In other words, the normal treatment for hemochromatosis is that your blood is taken on a frequent, regular basis just like you would donate blood for a blood bank. The process is simple, safe and inexpensive. Yes, it's a bit inconvenient and is mildly uncomfortable, but that's a very small price to pay for successful treatment.

Here's how it works. Usually an individual with hemochromatosis "gives" blood (sometimes weekly) until measures of iron stores are reduced to a safe level, and then maintenance donations are given on a less frequent schedule *throughout life.*

If anemia is also present, however, drugs in the form of iron chelators may also be prescribed by doctors.

Phlebotomies

The number of phlebotomies necessary to "de-iron" the body varies depending on the severity of the disease discovered at diagnosis. The target of the phlebotomies is to reduce the blood ferritin levels to the very low end of normal and then keep them there.

As stated, phlebotomies are usually needed periodically throughout life in addition to the initially frequent treatment necessary to at first bring iron down to a safe level within the body.[12]

When an individual is first identified as having iron overload hemochromatosis, usually one to two pints of blood (which contains iron locked away in the hemoglobin of red blood cells) are initially removed from the patient on a weekly basis until the iron stores drop to a normal level. Each pint of blood contains about 200-250 mg of iron, which is roughly the amount of extra iron absorbed by the intestines over a three month period of time.

Naturally the phlebotomy treatments (frequency and amount of blood removed) are individualized to each patient and take into account the age, sex, size, weight, and stage of hemochromatosis. However, at this rate of phlebotomy therapy, and taking into account

---

[12] Borch-Iohnsen, "Primary hemochromatosis and dietary iron (in Norwegian)," *Tidsskr Nor Laegeforen* (Norway) Oct 10 1997, 117(24) p 3506-7.

18

the amount of iron absorbed from the diet, patients undergoing two 500-milliliter phlebotomies per week will usually lose about 50 mg of iron per day, or about 18 grams per year. Usually a person loses about 25-50 micrograms of ferritin per liter of blood serum. On this particular topic, University of Utah researchers wrote:

> Massive iron stores of 20 to 30 grams can be normalized in 12 to 18 months of twice-weekly phlebotomy. Because the time-dosage toxic threshold of iron that results in irreversible organ damage is known, iron stores should be completed completely and quickly. Phlebotomy performed at a rate of less than 500 milliliters every month may be counterproductive, as the rate of iron absorption from the diet may exceed the rate of iron depletion.[13]

The entire sequence of blood lettings for hemochromatosis patients may take anywhere from several months to several years to remove much of the excess iron, but if a person is treated early they can look forward to an extended lifespan or completely normal life without any organ damage. You only need to look at two studies to get a feel for this:

- In 1976, one study of brain-syndrome patients with hemochromatosis found that those whose iron stores were depleted through phlebotomy or chelation lived an average of 63 months after diagnosis, while untreated patients survived an average of only 18 months.[14]

- In 1985, another study of 163 hemochromatosis patients found that those without cirrhosis or diabetes at the time of diagnosis and treatment lived a normal

[13] Edwards, C.Q.; Griffen, L.M.; Kushner, J.P. "Disorders of excess iron." *Hospital Practice* April 1991; 26(3):30-26.
[14] Bomford, A and Williams R. "Long term results of venesection therapy in idiopathic hemochromatosis." *Queensland J Med.* 1976; 45:611.

life expectancy. Of the hemochromatosis patients who underwent iron therapy, 92% were alive after 5 years, 76% after 10 years, 59% after 15 years and 49% after 20 years.[15]

Remember, after the iron levels in the body are reduced to normal, the condition has not disappeared. An individual has not been cured. A hemochromatosis patient still needs to undertake maintenance phlebotomy treatments four to six times each year to prevent a re-accumulation of iron.

This lifetime maintenance is recommended because otherwise, any individual with hereditary hemochromatosis who neglects the blood letting may become iron overloaded again in a few years time once again.

Now if the hemochromatosis condition has progressed to a stage where it has caused liver cirrhosis, the situation is more serious than there just being an accumulation of excess iron in the system. The statistics show that liver cancer – because of the iron promoting free radical activity - can occur in up to 30% of these patients, which is why those for risk of liver cancer should be periodically tested. Those who have suffered liver damage are also advised to see a good naturopath and nutritionist who can help support the liver.

Hemochromatosis that damages the pancreas can also result in diabetes mellitus while damage to other organs may cause heart problems, chronic fatigue, joint pain, loss of body hair, loss of libido and infertility or impotence. As previously stated, in some advanced cases of hemochromatosis, the patient may develop an enlarged liver, liver cirrhosis or spleen enlargement.

In addition to the phlebotomies, the conventional treatments for

---

[15] Niederau C, et al. "Survival and causes of death in cirrhotic and non-cirrhotic patients with primary hemochromatosis." *New England J. Med.* 1985; 313: 1256.

hemochromatosis also include chelation therapy and dietary restrictions for patients. To avoid liver damage, a hemochromatosis suffer will also usually be told to avoid alcohol.

Additionally, to avoid excessive iron uptake, smart doctors will advise sufferers to avoid taking vitamin C with meals. Vitamin C increases your uptake of dietary iron but many internists and family practitioners don't know about this, and thus fail to warn patients.

They do know to warn patients to avoid eating iron-rich foods such as breakfast cereals fortified with 100% of the RDA of iron, eating raw shellfish (such as clams, oysters and shrimp), and cooking with cast-iron cookware.

We'll cover all these dietary rules in a subsequent chapter of this book. We'll also cover the fact that a hemochromatosis patient might also choose to drink tea with meals in order to help block the uptake of iron from the foods they eat, and thereby delay the frequency of phlebotomies.

None of the natural treatments to help with hemochromatosis "cure" the condition or get rid of the need for phlebotomies. When effective, they only help delay the uptake or excess iron into your system, but phlebotomies are still necessary.

Although the standard medical treatment cannot cure the conditions associated with established hemochromatosis, it will help most of them. The main exception seems to be arthritis, which does not improve even after the excess iron is removed from the body.

Again, once normal iron levels are re-established for a hemochromatosis sufferer, they can be maintained by periodic blood removal (2 to 6 times a year depending on the individual). The treatment of phlebotomies, or blood donation, will prevent damage that would have been caused by excess iron accumulation in the body, and once again you must remember that this treatment is ongoing for life. Researchers have found that ordinary individuals who donated one pint of blood each year were less likely to have cardiac events than casual donors, and so it is presumed that frequent blood donations will help reduce the risk of cardiac events for hemochromatosis sufferers.

Chelation Therapy

Chelation therapy is also sometimes used in cases of hemochromatosis, though phlebotomies are the recommended first line procedure for removing excess iron from the body.

Let's discuss how chelation works…

In chelation therapy, you're hooked up with an IV solution containing a special chelating chemical agent that, together with other nutrients, circulates throughout all the blood vessels in your body. A chemical chelating agent in the solution grasps certain minerals – such as iron, lead, mercury, cadmium, manganese -- and then escorts most of these toxic metals out of your body through your kidneys as urine.

In chelation therapy, your body gets rid of all sorts of accumulated metallic pollutants (not just iron), radiation particles, and assorted foreign elements that tend to cause cellular breakdown. It's often referred to as a rejuvenating therapy in the natural health field because of all the benefits won through the removal of heavy metals from the body.

If chelation therapy is a second line way to attack the condition, the logical question to ask is, "When is chelation therapy preferred over phlebotomy?"

The answer is: when a hemochromatosis patient suffers from angina or bone marrow suppression. These individuals usually do better receiving intravenous infusions of EDTA or **deferoxamine**

(**Desferal**), both of which are excellent iron chelators. In cases of iron detoxification or transfusion dependent anemias, most doctors will use Desferal (deferoxamine) for iron chelation.

Remember, even if you'd like an "alternative therapy," doctors usually don't administer chelation for primary hemochromatosis because phlebotomy is the current standard procedure. Yes, iron stores are indeed depleted through chelation therapy, but at a much slower rate than through phlebotomy. The phlebotomies are recommended.

Today there are a variety of oral chelating agents available on the market, and even rectal suppositories of products like **Detoxamin** (www.detoxamin.com) that are used for chelation under a doctor's supervision.

You might want to ask your doctor to check into these various products and their capabilities if you want to try chelation therapy without the trouble of an intravenous drip. This is not a decision for you to make alone, as you cannot depend on alternative therapies for this condition, however much you may like them.

The big thing is to start removing the excess iron from the body, once diagnosed with hemochromatosis, and to prevent a further uptake of excess iron that will contribute to the condition. This means that it's best to eliminate high iron content foods from the diet (Not eliminating iron entirely) and to possibly consume various supplements or food that will bind dietary iron so that it's not available for uptake.

This is where the field of alternative medicine excels with its recommendations, so now on to the dietary recommendations for hemochromatosis patients.

4
THE BASIC HEMOCHROMATOSIS DIET

The main dietary rule to help manage hemochromatosis is simple – decrease your consumption of foods that are rich in iron content or which tend to increase your natural tendency to iron absorption. However, you must not totally avoid iron-containing foods *entirely* or you are likely to become sick, weak or ill. If you reduce all iron from your diet, you are likely to develop iron deficiency anemia. The second set of dietary rules is to eat foods that tend to bind iron in the gut or bloodstream, and thus help reduce your iron stores that way.

In other words, you can adjust your diet to reduce the amount of iron you consume. You should also stop eating the foods that chemically help improve iron absorption, or eat them at times other than when you are eating iron-rich foods. Lastly, you can eat foods that are known to help bind iron, which is particularly important when you are eating iron-rich meals.

Frequent phlebotomies (bloodletting) are the treatment of choice for hemochromatosis although they do not remove excess iron from body tissues. They only remove iron in the blood. Since your body needs iron to survive, when you are undergoing frequent phlebotomies you should eat a well balanced diet that indeed contains iron to keep up your strength, or it may be hard to continue your treatment. Thais is why you should not eliminate iron completely from the diet. If you do, you'll quickly become weak and your diet will be unbearable to maintain.

Hence, someone can try to go "cold turkey" and try to eliminate the foods from your diet that contain iron, but this isn't wise. Altering your diet in this way does not cure hemochromatosis or prevent hemochromatosis. Yes, you can cut down on the frequency of high iron foods, but you should not eliminate them entirely if you want to stay healthy, maintain your strength and the ability to recover from any of the damage already done by the condition.

Phlebotomies will help you lower your iron load gradually, and as long as you don't fight this tendency to reduce your iron load by always eating high iron foods, you'll gradually reduce your iron stores. The important thing is not to emphasize foods in the diet that contain concentrated amounts of highly absorbable iron.

Now ... can the basic hemochromatosis dietary rules really help you manage your condition? Can they help you protect your body from building up excess iron stores that will harm your internal organs?

Sure!

It's a well proven fact that various dietary rules can help individuals mange their iron levels. For instance, restrictive iron-deficient dietary changes, for an individual who is perfectly fine, can produce anemia in a very short period of time – in as little as 120 days. Special iron-rich diets can also produce a state of iron overload with symptoms appearing in as little as 60 days. Lowering cholesterol in the diet can produce dramatic changes as well.

So what's normal for dietary iron intake?

The RDA (recommended daily allowance) for iron is 10 mg/day for adult men and for post-menopausal women. For pre-menopausal women, the RDA is 15 mg/day.

Because the intestines of a hemochromatosis patient absorb more iron than usual and because they already have high iron stores when diagnosed with the condition, they should not exacerbate this problem by constantly favoring high iron foods. The iron absorption rates from food vary widely - from 1% to nearly 100% -- so the key is not to make a highly absorbable, high iron food a frequent, standard staple of the diet.

That's the dietary rule to follow. Know what foods are iron-rich and readjust your diet so that they are not the central core of your food consumption.

What are these iron rich foods?

Cutting Down on Iron Rich Foods

The iron rich foods are just what you'd expect – **red meats** (steak, beef liver, etc.), **poultry, fish** and **seafood** (including clams, oysters, shrimp, etc.).

These are the richest sources of dietary iron. The iron within meats is also problematical because it comes in a form (heme iron) that is more readily absorbed by the body than the iron found in plants.

Now, whether or not it's related to iron consumption, restricting the consumption of red meat has been shown in various studies to reduce the risk of contracting colon cancer.[16] This is something you can often remind yourself when you are trying to cut down on meat consumption, if you choose to do so.

As to seafood, the big rule for hemochromatosis patients is never to eat raw seafood (cooked seafood is okay) if you are suffering from

---

[16] Kampman E, et al. "Meat consumption, genetic susceptibility, and colon cancer risk." *Cancer Epid Biomarker Prev* 1999; 8:15-24.

liver damage because it's possible to cause fatal liver infections. Therefore, no raw oysters or clams – especially since they are extremely heavy with iron content.

One should also not drink alcohol if there has been any sort of liver damage as well. Alcohol consumption easily damages one's liver and if the liver is already weak, you don't want to further damage it. Moderate alcohol consumption usually doesn't pose a problem with iron absorption, but excessive alcohol consumption is associated with iron overload.

There are plant foods that are high in iron as well that you should make note of. These include **enriched and whole grain cereals and breads** (such as iron fortified breakfast cereals), **tofu, dry beans** and **peas** (black beans, kidney beans, lima beans, pinto beans, lentils, chickpeas, baked beans, etc.), and **dark green leafy vegetables** (spinach, collard greens, swiss chard etc.).

The iron in these foods is in a form that is not as well absorbed by the body as is the iron fond in meat, poultry, and fish (non-heme iron). Typically, only about 5% of the iron found in plant foods becomes available to the body through intestinal absorption versus 30-50% of the iron available from red meats.

Blackstrap molasses is another food also rich in iron.

Interestingly enough, there are also certain spices and garnishes that promote iron absorption from the diet. These include: **olive oil** and spices such as **anise, caraway, cumin, licorice** and **mint**. If you cook with these spices, you are encouraging iron absorption, so you might wish to look at any tendencies to use these in your food recipes to see whether you are contributing to the condition in this way.

Once again, strictly following these various rules does not prevent hemochromatosis. They only help you to manage the condition.

Are there any other related rules related to cooking and the diet that are relevant?

Yes -- **Avoid using cast iron or stainless steel cooking pots** because they will increase the amount of iron you absorb. If you cook food in iron pots, naturally you'll actually increase your consumption of free iron.

And remember -- no fortified processed foods, especially iron fortified breakfast cereals. Check your cereal boxes and grain-food boxes for their iron content. Fortified Raisin Bran cereal is usually a typical high iron cereal, but you have to check the label as its iron content varies by manufacturer.

Remember, strictly following these dietary rules does not prevent the disease. It only helps to manage the condition of hemochromatosis, and that's all.

Iron Content of Selected Vegan Foods

FOOD	AMOUNT	IRON (mg)
Soybeans, cooked	1 cup	8.8
Blackstrap molasses	2 Tbsp	7.0
Lentils, cooked	1 cup	6.6
Tofu	4 oz	0.7-6.6
Quinoa, cooked	1 cup	6.3
Kidney beans, cooked	1 cup	5.2
Chickpeas, cooked	1 cup	4.7
Lima beans, cooked	1 cup	4.5
Pinto beans, cooked	1 cup	4.5
Veggie burger, commercial	1 patty	1.1-4.5
Black-eyed peas, cooked	1 cup	4.3
Swiss chard, cooked	1 cup	4.0
Tempeh	1 cup	3.8
Black beans, cooked	1 cup	3.6
Bagel, enriched	3 oz	3.2
Turnip greens, cooked	1 cup	3.2
Prune juice	8 oz	3.0
Spinach, cooked	1 cup	2.9
Beet greens, cooked	1 cup	2.7
Tahini	2 Tbsp	2.6

Raisins	1/2 cup	2.2
Cashews	1/4 cup	2.0
Figs, dried	5 medium	2.0
Seitan	4 oz	2.0
Bok choy, cooked	1 cup	1.8
Bulgur, cooked	1 cup	1.7
Apricots, dried	10 halves	1.6
Potato	1 large	1.4
Soy yogurt	6 oz	1.4
Tomato juice	8 oz	1.4
Veggie hot dog	1 hot dog	1.4
Almonds	1/4 cup	1.3
Peas, cooked	1 cup	1.3
Green beans, cooked	1 cup	1.2
Kale, cooked	1 cup	1.2
Sesame seeds	2 Tbsp	1.2
Sunflower seeds	1/4 cup	1.2
Broccoli, cooked	1 cup	1.1
Brussels sprouts,cooked	1 cup	1.1
Millet, cooked	1 cup	1.0
Prunes	5 medium	1.0
Watermelon	1/8 medium	1.0

Sources: USDA Nutrient Database for Standard Reference, Release 12, 1998. Manufacturer's information.

Nutritional Supplements and Vitamin C

One of the biggest mistake people with hemochromatosis make is taking multi-vitamin/multi-mineral supplements that contain iron. They may have been taking a multi-vitamin/mineral supplement for years, and never give it a thought to see if it also contains iron. That's just adding fuel to the fire, so-to-speak. You can find many vitamin-mineral supplements that include iron, and this is one of the first things you should do if you have the condition. By all means continue taking a supplement that might help your health and protect your internal organs from damage, but just make sure that it doesn't contain iron.

Let's depart from our discussion of hemochromatosis and just talk about the condition of excess iron in the body (an iron overload), without it being hemochromatosis, and see what the topic suggests to us about meal servings.

In a recent study of elderly Americans,[17] 13% of the participants had high serum ferritin iron stores, which were defined as serum ferritin levels over 300 μg/L in men and over 200 μg/L in women. We're not talking about hemochromatosis with these figures, but just high iron stores.

Naturally, red meat consumption and the consumption of fruit or fruit juice (because of the vitamin C content, which we'll discuss below) were identified as powerful risk factors for accumulating these high iron stores.

Here's what the studies show: **people who consumed three or more servings of fruit/fruit juice a day had a much higher risk of high iron stores than those who consumed two servings a day**.

This gives us our first indication of how much fruit/fruit juice is TOO MUCH for a hemochromatosis patient. If these amounts of fruit consumption are too much for ordinary individuals because they lead to higher iron stores, they are certainly good guidelines as to what hemochromatosis patients should avoid!

In this study, it was also found that those who consumed more than four servings of red meat a weak had three times the risk of high iron stores than participants who ate four servings a week. However, in this study, eating light meats such as poultry and seafood, did not affect the risk which suggests that poultry, even with its high heme-iron content, is a preferable meat than beef in terms of iron uptake.

Once again, managing your diet for hemochromatosis is a matter of adjusting the frequency and quantity of your meat consumption rather than eliminating meats altogether. **You do not have to**

---

[17] *American Journal Clinical Nutrition*, December 2002 76:1375-1384.

eliminate your red meat consumption entirely when you have hemochromatosis; it's just that "less is better than more, and some is better than none."

In a Norwegian study of hemochromatosis patients who wished to reduce the frequency of phlebotomies by regulating their diet, the study concluded that the following foods should be avoided:

- Ascorbic acid-rich fruit juice (particularly when taken with meals)
- Ascorbic acid-rich fruit (particularly when taken with meals)
- Alcohol
- Meat (in limited quantities)

This Norwegian dietary study also suggested that hemochromatosis patients follow a diet rich in the following:

- Non-iron fortified bread and cereals (fiber)
- Fruits (non-ascorbic acid varieties)
- Fresh vegetables

The consumption of **whole grains** was also found to decrease the risk of accumulating high iron stores in the body. Those who consumed more than seven servings of whole grains per week had a 77% lower risk of developing high iron stores than those who did not eat whole grains. Researchers speculated that this association was due to the inhibitory effect of fiber on the absorption of non-heme iron, which we'll also discuss in time, so keep that fact in the back of your mind.

Now here's the major point I wanted to get to: one of the most significant risk factors for developing high ferritin levels was consuming iron-containing supplements, which brings us back to hemochromatosis again. Those individuals who consumed between 12 and 30 mg of iron a day, which is an amount commonly found in multivitamins, had the strongest risks of high iron stores.

The moral of this all?

First, as previously stated, **don't take a multivitamin, multi-mineral supplement that contains iron** if you suffer from hemochromatosis! If you are taking a multivitamin, go right now and check if the label contains iron. If so, it would be prudent to replace your supplement with an iron free brand. The least thing you want to be doing right now is supplementing with the mineral whose accumulation may kill you!

Another thing to do is **cut down on your total vitamin C consumption** that you get through supplements because vitamin C increases iron absorption. If you wish to continue taking vitamin C supplements, take it between meals on an empty stomach. In that way, it will not increase your dietary iron absorption.

Remember, you cannot and should not try to eliminate vitamin C entirely from your diet altogether either. That's another recipe for catastrophe. There are lots of reasons for this:

- Vitamin C is needed for many body process – a deficiency will cause scurvy.

- In particular, published research shows that vitamin C acts as an antioxidant against lipid peroxidation (fats spoiling) when the blood is iron rich.

- While vitamin C does improve the absorption of dietary iron, it is also required to move iron out of ferritin tissue stores, so it is needed to help remove iron out of your tissues naturally. In other words, if you don't have enough antioxidants such as vitamin C and E, the iron in ferritin tissues cannot be transferred onto transferrin plasmin.

Therefore you should not eliminate your intake of vitamin C when you have hemochromatosis. Rather, you should learn to be cognizant of it and not overdo your vitamin C consumption. That's where people make the error.

Many people who take a lot of supplements never add up the total amount of vitamin C they are ingesting on a daily basis. They do not realize that with all the supplements they are taking (usually people take them with meals), they may be ingesting several thousand milligrams of vitamin C that ends increasing iron absorption!

When one of my nutritional clients came to me with high iron in his blood, we added up the total amount of vitamin C he was taking on a daily basis through of all the supplements he was consuming, and found several thousand milligrams per day! Simply by cutting down on these supplements, we were able to cut down on his total iron absorption and return things to normal in a short period of time.

Once again, don't try to avoid vitamin C altogether. You can and should eat vitamin C-containing fruits and drink fruit juices, but do this away from meals that contain a high concentration of iron. Also, don't overdo your consumption of these foods or supplements, but limit them to two servings per day.

Vitamin C should not be avoided altogether because of its many benefits, including the fact that studies show vitamin C consumptions is associated with a decreased risk for heart disease, cancer, cataracts and other disorders associated with hemochromatosis. You can check into the Linus Pauling Foundation for more information on the many benefits of vitamin C.

In short, the two big supplement rules are:

1. Reduce your intake of vitamin C – supplements and fruit/fruit juices – with meals. Rather, take any fruits or juices containing vitamin C apart from meals.
2. Reduce your intake of iron supplements

If you follow these rules, you're doing a lot to limit your iron absorption and helping to reduce the frequency of phlebotomies, which most hemochromatosis patients complain about.

Are there other dietary rules to follow that can help?

That's what we're covering next...

5
FOODS THAT HELP BLOCK
IRON ABSORPTION

One of the best ways of lowering the amount of iron you absorb from food is to eat other substances at the same time which help to block its absorption. You can do this with little trouble by ingesting fiber and calcium with your meals.

Let's discuss calcium's role in blocking iron absorption first.

It's just a fact of science that **calcium interferes with iron absorption**, and therefore this is a strategy you can use when planning meals to help with hemochromatosis. That strategy could be as simple as drinking milk with your meals or eating other calcium rich foods at the same time.

The American Journal of Clinical Nutrition stated that if you eat 300 mg of calcium with a meal, you would reduce the amount of iron you normally absorb by 40%. Therefore, this is a simple way to help reduce the iron in your blood,[18] though once again it does not eliminate the need for phlebotomies.

---

[18] Hallberg L, "Does calcium interfere with iron absorption?" *Am J Clin Nutr* 1998 Jul; 68(1):3-4.

How do you obtain 300 mg of calcium with a meal?

Simple – just take a calcium supplement that contains 300 mg of elemental calcium, which you can easily determine is in the supplement by reading its label. Many multi-vitamins contain calcium (but not iron), and since they should usually be eaten with a meal (since this helps absorption), simply select a good supplement with calcium and eat it at every meal.

According to published scientific studies that took accurate measurements, the maximum amount of calcium that will inhibit iron absorption is around 300 mg with each meal, so you are looking for a supplement with that amount of calcium. In other words, if you take more than 300 mg of calcium with your meal, it won't cause any additional interference with iron absorption. Therefore, only 300 mg is necessary; taking more is of no benefit in terms of blocking or interfering with iron absorption.

Most calcium or multi-vitamin/mineral supplements tell you how much elemental calcium they provide on the label, so all you have to do is look at the label to see what it says.

If you don't even want to look at labels, the easiest way to provide about 300 mg of elemental calcium is to take one or two 1000-mg capsules of calcium citrate with every meal that contains iron. So if you plan on eating red meats with lots of iron, you would supplement your meal with a calcium tablet.

The reason I recommend 1000-mg calcium citrate capsules is because each one provides about 220 mg of elemental calcium. Other types of calcium and other calcium supplements will provide a different amount of calcium per capsule dosage, which you can usually read off the label.

The problem with calcium consumption is that it not a strategy that you can count on using forever. Some people become tolerant to calcium-induced, iron-absorption blockage after several months. In other words, this strategy may stop working over time as your body gets used to it, which means you have to test to see if it is working by having regular blood tests to monitor your iron levels. It is better to control your iron absorption by managing your diet than by taking supplements, but it is an excellent strategy anyway to take a multivitamin/mineral supplement with a meal, but making sure it contains a sufficient amount of calcium. However, its inclusion in a formula is not necessary.

As previously stated, drinking milk is also known to inhibit the absorption of iron. Part of the reason for this is because milk contains calcium, but another reason is because it contains lactoferrin, which is another substance that tends to bind iron. Many foods other than dairy products bind iron because of their ingredients, and the next biggest food group that works this way are the fibers.

Pectin, for instance, is a non-digestible fiber that binds tightly to non-heme iron, and is also used in special dietary supplements to help prevent the spread of cancer to other organs. In one small study of 13 patients with idiopathic hemochromatosis, their dietary iron absorption decreased by nearly half following a loading dose of 9 grams/m2 of pectin (about 15 grams for the average adult).[19] You can increase your intake of pectin by eating more carrots, cucumbers, celery, legumes (beans), peas and tomatoes. Eating raw carrots now and then, such as in salads, is a great way to do this.

Many other foods can help limit iron absorption because they bind to it or interfere with its uptake. A short list of such foods includes:

---

[19] Monnier L; Colette C; Ribot C; Mirouze J, "Intestinal handling of iron and calcium in idiopathic haemochromatosis: new data and therapeutic perspectives." *Annales de Biologie Animale, Biochimie, Biophysique,* 1979; 19(3B): 775-780.

- Milk and dairy products (cheese and yoghurt) because they contain lactoferrin in addition to calcium.

- Soluble fibers such as psyllium seed husks (Metamucil), guar gum, and the pectins also help to block iron (and other mineral) absorption.

- Antacids, eggs and soy are known to reduce the availability of dietary iron.

- Carbonates, oxalates, and phosphates are also iron blockers and the foods that contain them include, cranberries, rhubarb, spinach, and soda.

- **Phytic acid** (a component of whole grains and seeds such as sesame) binds to iron and other minerals in the gastric tract and help to limit iron availability; eating whole grain breads and cereals therefore helps bind dietary iron and reduce its absorption from foods.

- **Bioflavonoids** (found in berries, coffee, green tea, pine bark, *quercetin* and the rind of citrus fruits, particularly blueberry, cranberry, elderberry and grape seed) also tend to bind to iron and prevent its uptake into the body.

The benefit of eating foods rich with bioflavonoids and phytic acid is that if these substances don't bind to minerals in the digestive tract, they will get absorbed into the bloodstream. Once in the bloodstream, they will tend to bind to any free iron they find and thus act as iron chelators for the blood.

Therefore, just as we want to consume any vitamin C and fruits apart from meals, it's good to know that we maximize the iron chelation abilities of these other foods for the blood when these iron binders are consumed apart from meals.

Avoid Extra Manganese

While we're discussing the mineral calcium, a word about **manganese** and iron …

The absorption of iron in the body is actually dependent on the mineral manganese (Mn). Many minor iron-deficiency situations can actually be reversed by manganese supplements without any need for iron supplementation! Therefore, the presence of manganese in your nutritional supplements when you have hemochromatosis is not necessarily a good thing because it might help to increase your iron absorption.

Some research studies say that manganese supplementation can protect against the free radical damage from excess iron[20] and some sources claim that manganese lowers iron levels, but this is mostly a theoretical consideration that would only happen under unusual circumstances.

In actual clinical settings, you will rarely if ever see a patient's iron (ferritin) levels decline as a result of taking a manganese supplement, even when very high doses of manganese are taken on an ongoing basis. This is still a matter under study by researchers, however, nevertheless the issue is pertinent enough to bring to your attention.

The point is that if you wish to take a multivitamin supplement, take a good look at the label for its iron, calcium, vitamin C and manganese contents.

---

[20] *Free Radical Biology and Medicine,* 1992; 13: pp.115-20.

6
DRINKING TANNIN-RICH TEA TO BIND DIETARY IRON

Another option for reducing your iron absorption is drinking tea with each meal.

That's right – drinking tea!

A study in the British medical journal *Gut*[21] revealed that drinking **tannin-rich black teas** with meals can reduce your iron absorption, and thus tea drinking is of benefit to those with hemochromatosis.

In the study, a control group of individuals drank water with their meals. The other group drank tea with their meals. Researchers then measured the intestinal iron absorption for each group by studying the test subjects' blood figures for serum iron binding capacity and serum ferritin.

The results?

The average intestinal absorption of iron was 6.9% for patients consuming tea (without any additions such as milk or lemon)

---

[21] Kaltwasser JP, et al. "Clinical trial on the effect of regular tea drinking on iron accumulation in genetic haemochromatosis." *Gut* 1998; 43:699-704.

compared with 22.1% in those drinking water with meals.

This is a 69% reduction in iron absorption! Furthermore, over a one-year period, the increase in iron storage was reduced by about one-third compared with the control group. In short, there was a significant reduction in the iron absorption for the tea drinking group as compared to the water drinkers. If iron absorption can be slowed, it can reduce the need for more frequent phlebotomies.

In 1982 another study[22] was performed designed to determine the effect of various drinks on iron absorption. Test subjects were fed a standard meal consisting of a hamburger, string beans, mashed potatoes and water.

When **green tea** was substituted for the water, measurements showed that dietary iron absorption was reduced by 62%. Milk and beer seemed to have no effect on iron absorption in this study (a different finding than in other studies, as the milk would normally limit iron consumption), but **coffee** reduced iron absorption by 35%.

As one would expect, orange juice – because it contains vitamin C – had the opposite effect and actually increased iron absorption by 85%. We already know that vitamin C usually increases iron absorption, which is why hemochromatosis patients should limit their intake of vitamin C in nutritional supplements.

In another British study, the inhibition of iron uptake by drinking black tea was found to be 79-94%, peppermint tea 84%, pennyroyal 73%, cocoa 71%, vervain 59%, lime flower 52% and chamomile 47%.[23]

Black tea has the strongest ability to bind iron of all beverages, followed by coffee and then the herbal teas such as chamomile.

---

[22] Hallberg L, Rossander L. "Effect of different drinks on the absorption of non-heme iron from composite meals." *Hum Nutr Appl Nutr* 1982; 36:116-23.
[23] Hurrell RF, Reddy M, Cook JD. "Inhibition of non-haem iron absorption in man by polyphenolic-containing beverages." *Br J Nutr.* 1999; 81(4):289-295.

The logical strategy that falls out of these studies is to **drink coffee or tea with meals to slow your dietary iron uptake**. In delaying the absorption of iron, this makes it easier for hemochromatosis patients to manage their rate of iron absorption from foods.

Nevertheless, the frequency for phlebotomies is something that your doctor should still determine even if you choose this routine, and should not be something you choose yourself. Only a doctor can determine the best frequency of your blood donations. These strategies only have the possibility of helping to prolong the gap of time between which one needs to give blood, but whether they actually work in this way has to be confirmed by blood tests.

Because **green tea** was found to be a potent iron-chelating agent, some nutritionists even recommend that you consume green tea extracts when you have hemochromatosis. This is based on a study where an extract of green tea with a meal eaten by healthy women inhibited the absorption of non-heme iron (the form of iron found in plant foods, dairy products and iron supplements) by 26%.[24]

This is also a strategy you might consider, and based on studies, you'd want to be taking beverages or capsules that contain between 100-400 mg total polyphenols per serving in order to reduce iron absorption by 60-90%.

Two studies (Imai 1995 and Samman 2001) have shown reductions in serum ferritin and iron absorption when green tea or green tea extract is consumed, while other studies have shown no benefit at all. However, since green tea contains power anti-oxidants that demonstrate an iron chelating activity similar to the iron chelating drug desferoxamine used for hemochromatosis, and since some green teas can help you lose weight or contain potent anti-cancer agents (EGCG), drinking green tea (and black tea) should probably

---

[24] Samman S, Sandstrom B, Toft MB, et al. "Green tea or rosemary extract added to foods reduces nonheme-iron absorption." *Am J Clin Nutr* 2001; 73:607–12.

be adopted into one's lifestyle when they have hemochromatosis.

Actually, most people find that drinking tea seems to be a better and more enjoyable option than eating tea capsules, and it's the option encouraged when patients have hemochromatosis.

The time old thinking since Hippocrates is that it's usually better to manage health conditions through food rather than medicines whenever possible, and because tea drinking is so easy and proven versus taking supplements, it is the route that most nutritionists would recommend to slow your iron absorption.

7
SUPPLEMENTS THAT HELP BIND IRON
OR PROTECT YOUR INTERNAL ORGANS

In addition to drinking tea or eating special foods (or avoiding certain foods), yet another way to cut down on iron absorption is to consume various nutritional supplements that tend to bind iron in your system.

Of course you can attempt to do this naturally without supplements by drinking tannin-rich black (or green) teas or by eating special foods, and this is the dietary approach most often recommended to helping control your iron absorption. Adjusting your diet is a very simple strategy that usually costs very little or nothing at all, so that's the approach most nutritionists and naturopaths personally favor.

Various types of dietary fiber also tend to bind iron in the gut but the probably most commonly cited substance to this are calcium supplements. You don't need to take calcium supplements, but can simply increase your calcium intake by drinking milk or eating calcium rich foods such as cheese, yoghurt, sardines, dark leafy vegetables (ex. spinach, kale, turnips, collard greens) and soybeans. Although fortified orange juice and fortified cereals (which are sources of fiber) contain extra calcium, the orange juice also contains vitamin C which increases iron absorption, and cereals are fortified with the iron you are trying to reduce.

When we turn from natural dietary sources of binding iron in the digestive tract, it turns out that several other specialized substances have also been found to help treat iron overload. They work by either binding excess iron in the blood or drawing it out of tissues, or by inhibiting iron absorption in the gut. Along these lines, the two substances you should know about are IP-6 and lactoferrin.

IP-6 (Inositol Hexaphosphate)

The substance IP-6 (inositol hexaphosphate), also known as phytic acid, is well known as an iron binding supplement. IP-6 is a natural substance comprised of six phosphorus molecules and one molecule of inositol, which is a member of the B vitamin complex.

For years researchers ignored IP-6 because it impairs mineral absorption, but in our case that's exactly what we want. Its ability to bind to minerals makes it a very cheap and non-toxic form of iron chelation that can be done without a doctor's prescription, and it has some positive side benefits as a nutritional supplement as well, especially in the treatment of cancer (and cancer is often connected with hemochromatosis). It is used in natural cancer treatments because it binds iron, and cancer cells need a lot of iron to replicate DNA when they divide in order to survive.

Now there's a little bit of confusion about IP-6, or phytic acid. When you supplement with phytic acid, which is derived from rice bran extract, it will bind to iron and other minerals in your digestive tract when you take it with food. When you take it apart from meals, however, it will enter your bloodstream and bind to any free iron and other minerals in the blood,[25] and then be eliminated through the kidneys as urine.[26] You don't want to bind all your minerals, so there are problems in using this supplements.

---

[25] Phytic acid removes only excess or unbound minerals, not mineral ions already attached to proteins.

[26] [No authors listed] "Phytic acid: new doors open for a chelator." *Lancet,* 1987 Sept 19:2; 2(8560):664-6.

Previously we mentioned chelation therapy as a way of binding iron and escorting it out of your system. Researchers speculate that phytic acid's ability to bind to iron will help it someday replace intravenous chelation therapy with EDTA or desferrioxamine (Desferal). That's how good it is at sequestering iron, which can come in handy during an infection when you want to deny iron's availability to bacteria, which need it to grow and thrive.

You cannot just run out and start taking IP-6 carelessly. If you ever choose to design any nutritional supplement routine using the information provided such as this, always discuss things with your physician. They'll know how much you can take of any supplement, and will be able to monitor your condition to make sure you don't get into trouble. The problem is that if IP-6 supplements are taken for more than several months then fatigue can set in as a result of iron deficiency!

As to other dangers, women should never take phytic acid supplements during pregnancy since it will deprive the developing fetus from the minerals necessary for healthy growth. If someone with anemia takes phytic acid, they are also likely to feel weaker after the supplementation.

Some hemochromatosis patients take aspirin for their condition because aspirin produces a small loss of blood per day that consequently helps to control iron levels. However, you should never simultaneously use phytic acid with a daily aspirin regimen either.

Usually a three-month course of phytic acid will produce a quite noticeable amount of iron chelation, and for normal individuals prolonged daily supplementation may actually lead to iron-deficiency anemia. While anemic individuals who take phytic acid are likely to start feeling weak shortly after they begin consuming it, iron-overloaded individuals (such as hemochromatosis sufferers) are likely to feel increased energy.

As stated, a benefit of IP-6 is that it can help with cancer, which is one of the worries of hemochromatosis patients. IP-6 can more get into cancer cells to chelate iron than the pharmaceutical drugs designed to do so. So while I know of no studies done specifically on this, IP-6 supplementation might be one way for your doctor to help prevent liver cancer in advanced cases of hemochromatosis with liver damage. Discuss it with your doctor.

Regardless of its many benefits, remember that supplemental IP-6 may slow down the amount of iron being absorbed from the digestive tract, but only specially formulated drugs or blood loss can remove iron from the body.

Tsuno Food & Rice Company of Wakayama Japan is the only manufacturer of IP-6 in the world. Since any brand you purchase would ultimately come from this company, purchasing the least expensive brand at a store such as www.iherb.com is probably the way to get the best deal.

Lactoferrin

Lactoferrin, which is a glycoprotein found in milk (and whey protein), has also often been mentioned as a possible supplement to help bind iron, and is often used as a means to withhold iron from bacteria during infections.

Lactoferrin belongs to the family of biological entities called cytokines, which coordinate the body's cellular immune defenses that protect us from most infections, tumors and cancers. Cytokines also boost the activity of T-cells and stimulate production of immunoglobulins within our bodies. It helps inhibit microbes by depriving them of the iron needed for their growth.

Since hemochromatosis sufferers are subject to higher incidents of infection and possible cancers, and since it binds iron, these various properties make lactoferrin of great interest, including the fact that it is readily available as a nutritional supplement.

In particular, lactoferrin has the ability to bind 300 times more iron than serum transferrin. It binds iron in areas outside the bloodstream such as in the GI tract, mucous membranes and reproductive tissues. In studies, lactoferrin has also been found to remove free iron from synovial fluid aspirated from the joints of rheumatoid arthritic patients.[27]

Because of these properties, researchers have been working on producing recombinant human lactoferrin, which is indistinguishable from natural breast milk lactoferrin with respect to its iron binding properties, and it is now available.[28] Of course natural lactoferrin is available as well, but pharmaceutical firms cannot make money on natural supplements because they don't offer the possibility of patents. The whole idea behind producing a synthetic lactoferrin in the first place was to create a product that could become an additional seller besides the de-ironing pharmaceutical products already available.

The question this begs is whether hemochromatosis sufferers should supplement with lactoferrin for its various benefits. As of today, no studies have yet been done, so it's a matter for the researchers and doctors to ponder. You can ask your doctor about this possibility, and when studies are done it might soon be recommended as an addition to the standard medical protocols for hemochromatosis.

Supplements to Protect Your Internal Organs

---

[27] Guillen C, McInnes IB, Kruger H, Brock JH. "Iron, lactoferrin-and iron regulatory protein activity in the synovium; relative importance of iron loading and the inflammatory response." *Ann Rheum Dis* 1998; 57:309-14.
[28] Ward PP, Piddington CS, Cunningham GA, Zhou X, Wyatt RD, Conneely OM. "A system for production of commercial quantities of human lactoferrin, a broad spectrum natural antibiotic." *Biotechnology* 1995; 13:498-503.

Another large issue which arises is how to protect your body and its internal organs through supplements if they are susceptible to iron overdose. While you can change your diet and eat various supplements to help bind iron and reduce it in your system, the question arises whether you can do anything to protect specific organs highly susceptible to excess iron damage.

There are two approaches to this using nutritional supplements. The first is to try to chelate out of your body the excess iron that has built up within your tissues so that it doesn't oxidize and cause organ damage. The second approach is to optimize your antioxidant intake in order to protect your body from the destructive effects of excess iron. This means ingesting more of the *right kind* of antioxidants with iron protective properties.

While your heart, brain and pancreas are all typically at risk with hemochromatosis, the one organ you should particularly focus on is the liver because it is often severely damaged through iron overload diseases. What can you do to protect your liver if you have hemochromatosis?

It turns out that there are three ingredients commonly found within nutritional supplements that have traditionally been used to protect the liver, and which have also been shown to protect the body against excessive iron levels. This is a great coincidence, and when selecting a liver protecting or support formula we should be looking for these ingredients on the label. The following top liver protectors tend to bind or reduce iron in your system:

> Milk Thistle
> Alpha Lipoic Acid
> Curcumin

Milk Thistle, and its active ingredient Silymarin, have been shown in countless research studies to help protect the liver and gallbaldder, and since the liver is often damaged in hemochromatosis you might consider taking a liver support supplement that contains this as an active ingredient. Milk Thistle and Silymarin are a staple in most liver protectant supplements and liver strengthening nutritional formulas because they help prevent the fibrosis of liver scarring and liver failure, so a suitable supplement containing these ingredients is usually not hard to find. The interesting thing is that they have also been shown to have strong iron chelation properties!

For instance, 140 mg of silybin (the main component of silymarin) when taken by hemochromatosis patients in a test meal containing about 14 mg of non-heme iron, was shown to reduce iron absorption by over 40% (Hutchinson 2010). Furthermore, when silymarin was used (140 mg three times per day) in conjunction with the injectable iron chelator desferoxamine, the result was more effective reductions in serum ferritin than desferoxamine alone for beta-thalassemia patients (Gharagozloo 2009).

Alpha lipoic acid, a well known antioxidant, is the second item on our list of substances known to both protect the liver and protect against iron metabolism. It is also used in hundreds of nutritional formulas because it is both a water and fat soluble antioxidant, and has been definitively shown to act as a protector against free radicals and help with countless disease conditions. It helps protect you in cases of heart disease, diabetes and liver dysfunction. You want to ideally see this in any liver or other organ protective formula as well.

What is of interest to us that alpha lipoic acid (in its reduced form, dihydrolipoic acid) was specifically shown to protect neurons against iron-catalyzed oxidative damage (Lovell 2003). Furthermore, in an interesting study R-alpha lipoic acid was fed to older rats with age-related accumulation of iron in their cerebral cortex. Following two weeks of supplementation, the study found that the iron levels dropped to those indicative of younger rats (Suh 2005). As an supplement to help protect the liver, combat iron-induced free radical damage, help reduce iron and provide other benefits, alpha lipoic acid should be added to our list. Usually alpha lipoic acid or NAC (N-acetyl-cysteine) are usually major ingredients in liver detoxification or support formulas.

Coenzyme Q10, also known as CoQ10, is one of those substances also known to help alleviate the symptoms of many existing health conditions, and has a tendency to act as a chelating agent for metals such as iron. This is especially important for heart health which may be affected in cases of hemochromatosis. When a nutritionist thinks of cardiac health supplements, they always think of CoQ10, especially if someone is taking cholesterol lowering medications.

Quercetin, which was previously mentioned in passing, is a naturally occurring plant molecule that has the ability to bind to free iron atoms, and is known to protect against *kidney damage* associated with acute iron overload. In lab studies, animals who supplemented with quercetin were able to avoid liver injury from long term iron exposure. Quercetin is usually found in allergy supplements and in resveratrol supplements that people normally consume in interests of blood sugar control (diabetes) and *longevity*. This is a iron binding supplement to consider if you have weak kidneys, are prone to allergies or hayfever, or there is a tendency to diabetes in the family.

Cranberry and pomegranate extracts are rich in polyphenols, and have been shown to have strong iron-chelating abilities. Since cranberry juice is a well known home remedy for urinary tract infections, you might consider this as an addition to your diet if you commonly suffer from urinary tract infections. Why? Because it will also tend protect your kidneys from excess iron accumulation at the same time.

The key to altering your diet, or selecting supplements for their protective nature, is not simply to consumer everything (which would be far too expensive), but to find those common indications where logical dietary changes and supplementation might help multiple problems at once. In the case of quercetin, if you have hemochromatosis AND allergies then it is logical to consider this supplement. If you suffer from frequent urinary tract infections and hemochromatosis, you would consider cranberry juice. If heart disease or cardiac events run in your family, then you would consider CoQ10 as an iron protective supplement. If cancer or brain conditions such as Alzheimer's or Parkinson's are a family tendency, then you would consider drinking **green tea** as a dietary habit since it contains the powerful molecule **EGCG** that crosses the blood brain barrier and helps chelate iron out of the body. Scientists have proposed using EGCG as an alternative to commercial iron chelators, and it has been used to treat thalassemia where iron accumulates in the body due to excessive numbers of blood transfusions.

Lastly, the common spice turmeric contains **curcumin**, which has active components proven to be great antioxidants and iron chelators. Curcumin also helps to protect your immune system, maintain a healthy digestive tract, improve skin appearance, and support healthy joint function (which often gets attacked in hemochromatosis). It helps prevent pancreatic cancer and treats pancreatitis, and the pancreas is often severely damaged by hemochromatosis. If there is a tendency to diabetes in the family or pancreatic problems, this supplement is one to consider. Day after day, researchers are discovering more and more benefits to this simple compound.

For instance, a variety of studies suggest that curcumin can greatly reduce liver damage that is associated with iron-caused lipid peroxidation, iron-catalyzed oxidative damage of DNA, and free-radical damage due to iron found in the amyloid plaques of Alzheimer's disease. In mice with beta-thalassemia, the curcuminoids of curcumin were found to chelate iron out of the blood and reduce cardiac iron deposits caused by high-iron diets. It has even been found to reduce iron-associated lipid peroxidation when combined with the IV chelator deferiprone.

If you have hemochromatosis, you should know of the tendency for liver disease affecting those who have the condition. While you can reduce your intake of dietary iron through wiser eating habits and try to bind it through various foods supplements, you might consider taking a liver support formula that contains these and other detoxification ingredients that together synergistically offer multifaceted liver and joint protection, and can help protect other internal organs as well that are often affected by the condition.

There are many such formulas on the market, such as Jarrow's "Liver PF" formula, "Pure Encapsulations LVR Formula," Now brand's "Liver Detoxifier & Regenerator" and others which contains alpha lipoic acid, silymarin and other liver protectorants, in amounts sufficient to help protect the liver from damage.

This is a very important strategy when you have hemochromatosis. You should consider what organs tend to be weak in your family line, assume you also have those "weak link" genetics, and then supplement according to those indications. Naturally you would take supplements to protect and support organs that have already been damaged due to hemochromatosis, but the big takeaway is to think about the tendencies within your family, assume you have similar genetics and therefore similar organ weaknesses, and then use protective supplements as a preventive. This nutritional/naturopathic approach is logical, simple and cheaper than taking every iron binding or antioxidant supplement under the sun, which can actually be a harmful strategy.

8
ASPIRIN AND EXERCISE
AS SUFFICENT PROTOCOLS?

Most people know that some doctors will recommend taking an aspirin a day to prevent heart attacks and strokes. However, taking an aspirin every day causes a small amount of blood loss via the digestive tract. It's a tiny amount on the order of about a tablespoon per day.

This blood loss results in iron loss. Therefore, by ingesting a baby aspirin per day, Raymond Hohl, M.D. (an assistant professor of internal medicine and pharmacology) at the University of Iowa says that this strategy may help to control your iron stores. But remember, taking an aspirin a day also poses other significant dangers, such as inducing iron-deficiency anemia.[29]

Countless health articles also warn about dangers in taking aspirin on a daily basis, despite all the pharmaceutical company sponsored positive statements, therefore you should really think deeply about this strategy if it is recommended to you as a means of helping you to control hemochromatosis. You should read as many articles possible

---

[29] Bankhead C. "In assessing anemia, doctors must decipher role of iron deficiency." *Med Tribune Clin Focus* 1997; Mar, 20:24.

on the dangers od daily aspirin ingestion and also look up the number of individuals sent to the hospital each year due to aspirin usage before you decide to go on any long term aspirin regimen.

Rather than by ingesting aspirin, a person also loses about 1 mg of iron through sweat[30] caused by exercising. Many men and women who engage in regular, intensive exercise such as jogging, competitive swimming, and cycling end up having marginal or inadequate iron status, so exercising may be a natural way to help reduce your iron stores, too. However, you cannot depend on this alone, so don't take this as a cure for hemochromatosis!

The possible explanations for this iron deficiency in athletes include increased gastrointestinal blood loss after running (such as the blood loss caused by aspirin) and a greater turnover of red blood cells. Also, red blood cells within the foot often rupture while running.

In any case, this is something that researchers must study before doctors will recommend exercise as a way to help control iron overload. There is a definite tie-in between the tendency of exercise to reduce your iron stores, but one absolutely cannot depend on this route alone to manage your hemochromatosis just as you should not depend on aspirin alone to reduce your iron status either.

---

[30] Vellar OD. "Studies on sweat losses of nutrients." *Scand J Clin Lab Invest* 1968; 21:157-67.

9
SUMMARY

If hemochromatosis is discovered early before major organ damage has been done, with phlebotomies one can manage your iron levels, restore them to normal, and you are likely to live a very long life.

Nevertheless, regular blood donations (phlebotomy) do not cure the problem of hemochromatosis. The body has a tendency, for whatever reason, to absorb excessive amounts of iron, and so you will have to learn how to manage that condition. You will certainly need to continue donating blood throughout life, on a regular basis, to prevent your iron stores from building to dangerous levels.

The big question is whether you can slow the frequency of troublesome phlebotomies. This can only be done by managing your diet, and yet you do not want to go to dietary extremes and reduce your dietary iron intake to zero. That will lead to health issues, too, such as anemia.

Even so, a number of established dietary rules will help reduce your iron intake, and thus possibly reduce your doctor's recommendation for the frequency of phlebotomies once the basic condition is under control. Just following these simple dietary rules constitutes the basic "Hemochromatosis Diet." You certainly do not need any special "hemochromatosis cookbook" for hemochromatosis friendly meals when you simply follow these guidelines (that avoid iron), which include:

- Reducing the consumption of red meats (beef, lamb, turkey, etc.) and seafood that contain highly absorbable heme iron, and reducing the intake of iron fortified foods such as breakfast cereals.

- Reducing the consumption of fruits and juices with high-iron meals when they contain high levels of vitamin C, and eat them only between meals. Eat at most two servings per day.

- You should also reduce the intake of vitamin C supplements when simultaneously eating high iron content foods because vitamin C will increase your iron absorption. You don't want to stop taking vitamin C, you just want to stop taking vitamin C when you are also eating high iron content foods at the same time.

- Stop cooking with iron cookware.

- If you work in an industrial environment that exposes you to high levels of iron (such as working with iron oxide pigments), then take appropriate protective measures such as wearing a face mask.

- Eliminate iron and manganese supplements from the diet. Switch to multi-vitamin/mineral supplements that have no iron since you are already getting enough from the diet.

- When you eat red meats or seafood, you might consider eating foods at the same time which help to bind dietary iron such as milk, dairy products, soluble fibers, antacids, eggs, soy, cranberries, rhubarb, spinach, whole grain breads and cereals, and blueberries. Fiber and calcium are especially important.

- Drink green or black tea (tannin-rich tea) with meals to help bind the dietary iron in your meals.

- Take calcium supplements with meals to help bind iron (or green tea capsules), or simply eat yoghurt, drink milk or ingest some other form of dietary calcium at the same time.

- Adjust your cooking recipes that use spices such as anise, caraway, cumin, licorice and mint that increase iron uptake and substitute other herbs instead.

- Check with your doctor about the possibilities of using IP-6, and substances like lactoferrin, to bind iron when necessary. The use of such expensive supplements is not usually necessary or recommended. Just by changing your diet in little ways, you can greatly reduce your iron intake dramatically and need not use any special supplements at all.

- Take supplements that can help protect your liver (silymarin, alpha lipoic acid, curcumin, etc.), heart (COQ10), pancreas (quercetin, curcumin, alpha lipoic acid), kidneys, brain (EGCG, green tea extract, etc.) and other internal organs often harmed or damaged by hemochromatosis. If the supplement both supports the protection of the organ in general, and also serves as an iron binder, chelator or inhibitor, it can perform double duty and is especially desirable in any formulation. Consider any organs that have already been harmed by your condition, or your family genetics when making a supplement decision.

There are a variety of other infrequent sources of iron exposure (and ingestion) we have not covered such as inhaling amosite, crocidolite, or tremolite asbestos; mining iron ore; welding; grinding steel; painting with iron oxide powder or working with iron oxides in general. If you work in an iron rich environment, **wearing a face mask** will help cut down on iron absorption into your bloodstream. Even cigarette smoking is a source of iron for the body because about 1-2 μg iron are inhaled per cigarette pack, so cutting down on cigarette smoking will reduce youriero0n absorption as well.

All these things contribute to iron ingestion and thus iron overload. The point is to decrease your exposure to iron in any way you can but remember not to totally eliminate iron from your diet. Let the phlebotomies do their work, and work with your doctor and nutritionist/naturopath to help regenerate any damage to organs already done because of iron overload. The field of nutritional health offers many supplements that can help restore organs to tip top condition.

If you need more help or have more questions about hemochromatosis, you can turn to the following organizations that provide more information on this condition.

RELEVANT ORGANIZATIONS

American Hemochromatosis Society Inc.
4044 West Lake Mary Boulevard
Unit #104, PMB 416
Lake Mary, FL 32746–2012
Phone: 1–888–655–IRON (4766) or 407–829–4488
Fax: 407–333–1284
Email: mail@americanhs.org
Internet: www.americanhs.org

American Liver Foundation (ALF)
75 Maiden Lane
Suite 603
New York, NY 10038–4810
Phone: 1–800–465–4837,
1–888–443–7872,
or 212–668–1000
Fax: 212–483–8179
Email: info@liverfoundation.org
Internet: www.liverfoundation.org

Iron Disorders Institute Inc.
P.O. Box 2031
Greenville, SC 29602
Phone: 1–888–565–IRON (4766) or 864–292–1175

Fax: 864–292–1878
Email: publications@irondisorders.org
Internet: www.irondisorders.org

National Organization for Rare Disorders Inc.

55 Kenosia Avenue
P.O. Box 1968
Danbury, CT 06813–1968
Phone: 1–800–999–6673 or 203–744–0100
Fax: 203–798–2291
Email: orphan@rarediseases.org
Internet: www.rarediseases.org